INCIDENT / ACCIDENT FORM

CW00386261

| INCIDENT DATE: | INCIDENT TIME: |
| LOCATION: | DATE & TIME REPORTED: |

PERSON INJURED / INVOLVED: – EMPLOYEE – VISITOR – GENERAL PUBLIC – CONTRACTOR – OTHER

FULL NAME:

ADDRESS:

| PHONE: | EMAIL: |

DETAILS OF INCIDENT/ACCIDENT

NATURE & EXTENT OF INJURIES:

WHAT ACTION WAS TAKEN: – FIRST AID – AMBULANCE CALLED – HOSPITAL – POLICE – OTHER (PLEASE SPECIFY)

WITNESS(ES)

| NAME: | CONTACT: |
| NAME: | CONTACT: |

ACTIONS WHICH COULD HAVE PREVENTED THE INCIDENT

FORM COMPLETED BY:	DATE:
APPROVED BY:	POSITION:
SIGNATURE:	DATE:

INCIDENT / ACCIDENT FORM

INCIDENT DATE:	INCIDENT TIME:
LOCATION:	DATE & TIME REPORTED:

PERSON INJURED / INVOLVED: - EMPLOYEE - VISITOR - GENERAL PUBLIC - CONTRACTOR - OTHER

FULL NAME:

ADDRESS:

PHONE:	EMAIL:

DETAILS OF INCIDENT/ACCIDENT

NATURE & EXTENT OF INJURIES:

WHAT ACTION WAS TAKEN: - FIRST AID - AMBULANCE CALLED - HOSPITAL - POLICE - OTHER (PLEASE SPECIFY)

WITNESS(ES)

NAME:	CONTACT:
NAME:	CONTACT:

ACTIONS WHICH COULD HAVE PREVENTED THE INCIDENT

FORM COMPLETED BY:	DATE:
APPROVED BY:	POSITION:
SIGNATURE:	DATE:

INCIDENT / ACCIDENT FORM

INCIDENT DATE:	INCIDENT TIME:
LOCATION:	DATE & TIME REPORTED:

PERSON INJURED / INVOLVED: - EMPLOYEE - VISITOR - GENERAL PUBLIC - CONTRACTOR - OTHER

FULL NAME:

ADDRESS:

PHONE:	EMAIL:

DETAILS OF INCIDENT/ACCIDENT

NATURE & EXTENT OF INJURIES:

WHAT ACTION WAS TAKEN: - FIRST AID - AMBULANCE CALLED - HOSPITAL - POLICE - OTHER (PLEASE SPECIFY)

WITNESS(ES)

NAME:	CONTACT:
NAME:	CONTACT:

ACTIONS WHICH COULD HAVE PREVENTED THE INCIDENT

FORM COMPLETED BY:	DATE:
APPROVED BY:	POSITION:
SIGNATURE:	DATE:

INCIDENT / ACCIDENT FORM

INCIDENT DATE:	INCIDENT TIME:
LOCATION:	DATE & TIME REPORTED:

PERSON INJURED / INVOLVED: – EMPLOYEE – VISITOR – GENERAL PUBLIC – CONTRACTOR – OTHER

FULL NAME:

ADDRESS:

PHONE:	EMAIL:

DETAILS OF INCIDENT/ACCIDENT

NATURE & EXTENT OF INJURIES:

WHAT ACTION WAS TAKEN: – FIRST AID – AMBULANCE CALLED – HOSPITAL – POLICE – OTHER (PLEASE SPECIFY)

WITNESS(ES)

NAME:	CONTACT:
NAME:	CONTACT:

ACTIONS WHICH COULD HAVE PREVENTED THE INCIDENT

FORM COMPLETED BY:	DATE:
APPROVED BY:	POSITION:
SIGNATURE:	DATE:

INCIDENT / ACCIDENT FORM

INCIDENT DATE:	INCIDENT TIME:
LOCATION:	DATE & TIME REPORTED:

PERSON INJURED / INVOLVED: – EMPLOYEE – VISITOR – GENERAL PUBLIC – CONTRACTOR – OTHER

FULL NAME:

ADDRESS:

PHONE:	EMAIL:

DETAILS OF INCIDENT/ACCIDENT

NATURE & EXTENT OF INJURIES:

WHAT ACTION WAS TAKEN: – FIRST AID – AMBULANCE CALLED – HOSPITAL – POLICE – OTHER (PLEASE SPECIFY)

WITNESS(ES)

NAME:	CONTACT:
NAME:	CONTACT:

ACTIONS WHICH COULD HAVE PREVENTED THE INCIDENT

FORM COMPLETED BY:	DATE:
APPROVED BY:	POSITION:
SIGNATURE:	DATE:

INCIDENT / ACCIDENT FORM

INCIDENT DATE:	INCIDENT TIME:
LOCATION:	DATE & TIME REPORTED:

PERSON INJURED / INVOLVED: – EMPLOYEE – VISITOR – GENERAL PUBLIC – CONTRACTOR – OTHER

FULL NAME:

ADDRESS:

PHONE:	EMAIL:

DETAILS OF INCIDENT/ACCIDENT

NATURE & EXTENT OF INJURIES:

WHAT ACTION WAS TAKEN: – FIRST AID – AMBULANCE CALLED – HOSPITAL – POLICE – OTHER (PLEASE SPECIFY)

WITNESS(ES)

NAME:	CONTACT:
NAME:	CONTACT:

ACTIONS WHICH COULD HAVE PREVENTED THE INCIDENT

FORM COMPLETED BY:	DATE:
APPROVED BY:	POSITION:
SIGNATURE:	DATE:

INCIDENT / ACCIDENT FORM

INCIDENT DATE:	INCIDENT TIME:
LOCATION:	DATE & TIME REPORTED:

PERSON INJURED / INVOLVED: - EMPLOYEE - VISITOR - GENERAL PUBLIC - CONTRACTOR - OTHER

FULL NAME:

ADDRESS:

PHONE:	EMAIL:

DETAILS OF INCIDENT/ACCIDENT

NATURE & EXTENT OF INJURIES:

WHAT ACTION WAS TAKEN: - FIRST AID - AMBULANCE CALLED - HOSPITAL - POLICE - OTHER (PLEASE SPECIFY)

WITNESS(ES)

NAME:	CONTACT:
NAME:	CONTACT:

ACTIONS WHICH COULD HAVE PREVENTED THE INCIDENT

FORM COMPLETED BY:	DATE:
APPROVED BY:	POSITION:
SIGNATURE:	DATE:

INCIDENT / ACCIDENT FORM

INCIDENT DATE:	INCIDENT TIME:
LOCATION:	DATE & TIME REPORTED:

PERSON INJURED / INVOLVED: – EMPLOYEE – VISITOR – GENERAL PUBLIC – CONTRACTOR – OTHER

FULL NAME:

ADDRESS:

PHONE:	EMAIL:

DETAILS OF INCIDENT/ACCIDENT

NATURE & EXTENT OF INJURIES:

WHAT ACTION WAS TAKEN: – FIRST AID – AMBULANCE CALLED – HOSPITAL – POLICE – OTHER (PLEASE SPECIFY)

WITNESS(ES)

NAME:	CONTACT:
NAME:	CONTACT:

ACTIONS WHICH COULD HAVE PREVENTED THE INCIDENT

FORM COMPLETED BY:	DATE:
APPROVED BY:	POSITION:
SIGNATURE:	DATE:

INCIDENT / ACCIDENT FORM

INCIDENT DATE:	INCIDENT TIME:
LOCATION:	DATE & TIME REPORTED:

PERSON INJURED / INVOLVED: – EMPLOYEE – VISITOR – GENERAL PUBLIC – CONTRACTOR – OTHER

FULL NAME:

ADDRESS:

PHONE:	EMAIL:

DETAILS OF INCIDENT/ACCIDENT

NATURE & EXTENT OF INJURIES:

WHAT ACTION WAS TAKEN: – FIRST AID – AMBULANCE CALLED – HOSPITAL – POLICE – OTHER (PLEASE SPECIFY)

WITNESS(ES)

NAME:	CONTACT:
NAME:	CONTACT:

ACTIONS WHICH COULD HAVE PREVENTED THE INCIDENT

FORM COMPLETED BY:	DATE:
APPROVED BY:	POSITION:
SIGNATURE:	DATE:

INCIDENT / ACCIDENT FORM

INCIDENT DATE:	INCIDENT TIME:
LOCATION:	DATE & TIME REPORTED:

PERSON INJURED / INVOLVED: – EMPLOYEE – VISITOR – GENERAL PUBLIC – CONTRACTOR – OTHER

FULL NAME:

ADDRESS:

PHONE:	EMAIL:

DETAILS OF INCIDENT/ACCIDENT

NATURE & EXTENT OF INJURIES:

WHAT ACTION WAS TAKEN: – FIRST AID – AMBULANCE CALLED – HOSPITAL – POLICE – OTHER (PLEASE SPECIFY)

WITNESS(ES)

NAME:	CONTACT:
NAME:	CONTACT:

ACTIONS WHICH COULD HAVE PREVENTED THE INCIDENT

FORM COMPLETED BY:	DATE:
APPROVED BY:	POSITION:
SIGNATURE:	DATE:

INCIDENT / ACCIDENT FORM

INCIDENT DATE:	INCIDENT TIME:
LOCATION:	DATE & TIME REPORTED:

PERSON INJURED / INVOLVED: - EMPLOYEE - VISITOR - GENERAL PUBLIC - CONTRACTOR - OTHER

FULL NAME:

ADDRESS:

PHONE:	EMAIL:

DETAILS OF INCIDENT/ACCIDENT

NATURE & EXTENT OF INJURIES:

WHAT ACTION WAS TAKEN: - FIRST AID - AMBULANCE CALLED - HOSPITAL - POLICE - OTHER (PLEASE SPECIFY)

WITNESS(ES)

NAME:	CONTACT:
NAME:	CONTACT:

ACTIONS WHICH COULD HAVE PREVENTED THE INCIDENT

FORM COMPLETED BY:	DATE:
APPROVED BY:	POSITION:
SIGNATURE:	DATE:

INCIDENT / ACCIDENT FORM

INCIDENT DATE:	INCIDENT TIME:
LOCATION:	DATE & TIME REPORTED:

PERSON INJURED / INVOLVED: – EMPLOYEE – VISITOR – GENERAL PUBLIC – CONTRACTOR – OTHER

FULL NAME:

ADDRESS:

PHONE:	EMAIL:

DETAILS OF INCIDENT/ACCIDENT

NATURE & EXTENT OF INJURIES:

WHAT ACTION WAS TAKEN: – FIRST AID – AMBULANCE CALLED – HOSPITAL – POLICE – OTHER (PLEASE SPECIFY)

WITNESS(ES)

NAME:	CONTACT:
NAME:	CONTACT:

ACTIONS WHICH COULD HAVE PREVENTED THE INCIDENT

FORM COMPLETED BY:	DATE:
APPROVED BY:	POSITION:
SIGNATURE:	DATE:

INCIDENT / ACCIDENT FORM

INCIDENT DATE:	INCIDENT TIME:
LOCATION:	DATE & TIME REPORTED:

PERSON INJURED / INVOLVED: – EMPLOYEE – VISITOR – GENERAL PUBLIC – CONTRACTOR – OTHER

FULL NAME:

ADDRESS:

PHONE:	EMAIL:

DETAILS OF INCIDENT/ACCIDENT

NATURE & EXTENT OF INJURIES:

WHAT ACTION WAS TAKEN: – FIRST AID – AMBULANCE CALLED – HOSPITAL – POLICE – OTHER (PLEASE SPECIFY)

WITNESS(ES)

NAME:	CONTACT:
NAME:	CONTACT:

ACTIONS WHICH COULD HAVE PREVENTED THE INCIDENT

FORM COMPLETED BY:	DATE:
APPROVED BY:	POSITION:
SIGNATURE:	DATE:

INCIDENT / ACCIDENT FORM

INCIDENT DATE:	INCIDENT TIME:
LOCATION:	DATE & TIME REPORTED:

PERSON INJURED / INVOLVED: - EMPLOYEE - VISITOR - GENERAL PUBLIC - CONTRACTOR - OTHER

FULL NAME:

ADDRESS:

PHONE:	EMAIL:

DETAILS OF INCIDENT/ACCIDENT

NATURE & EXTENT OF INJURIES:

WHAT ACTION WAS TAKEN: - FIRST AID - AMBULANCE CALLED - HOSPITAL - POLICE - OTHER (PLEASE SPECIFY)

WITNESS(ES)

NAME:	CONTACT:
NAME:	CONTACT:

ACTIONS WHICH COULD HAVE PREVENTED THE INCIDENT

FORM COMPLETED BY:	DATE:
APPROVED BY:	POSITION:
SIGNATURE:	DATE:

INCIDENT / ACCIDENT FORM

INCIDENT DATE:	INCIDENT TIME:
LOCATION:	DATE & TIME REPORTED:

PERSON INJURED / INVOLVED: - EMPLOYEE - VISITOR - GENERAL PUBLIC - CONTRACTOR - OTHER

FULL NAME:

ADDRESS:

PHONE:	EMAIL:

DETAILS OF INCIDENT/ACCIDENT

NATURE & EXTENT OF INJURIES:

WHAT ACTION WAS TAKEN: - FIRST AID - AMBULANCE CALLED - HOSPITAL - POLICE - OTHER (PLEASE SPECIFY)

WITNESS(ES)

NAME:	CONTACT:
NAME:	CONTACT:

ACTIONS WHICH COULD HAVE PREVENTED THE INCIDENT

FORM COMPLETED BY:	DATE:
APPROVED BY:	POSITION:
SIGNATURE:	DATE:

INCIDENT / ACCIDENT FORM

INCIDENT DATE:	INCIDENT TIME:
LOCATION:	DATE & TIME REPORTED:

PERSON INJURED / INVOLVED: – EMPLOYEE – VISITOR – GENERAL PUBLIC – CONTRACTOR – OTHER

FULL NAME:

ADDRESS:

PHONE:	EMAIL:

DETAILS OF INCIDENT/ACCIDENT

NATURE & EXTENT OF INJURIES:

WHAT ACTION WAS TAKEN: – FIRST AID – AMBULANCE CALLED – HOSPITAL – POLICE – OTHER (PLEASE SPECIFY)

WITNESS(ES)

NAME:	CONTACT:
NAME:	CONTACT:

ACTIONS WHICH COULD HAVE PREVENTED THE INCIDENT

FORM COMPLETED BY:	DATE:
APPROVED BY:	POSITION:
SIGNATURE:	DATE:

INCIDENT / ACCIDENT FORM

INCIDENT DATE:	INCIDENT TIME:
LOCATION:	DATE & TIME REPORTED:

PERSON INJURED / INVOLVED: – EMPLOYEE – VISITOR – GENERAL PUBLIC – CONTRACTOR – OTHER

FULL NAME:

ADDRESS:

PHONE:	EMAIL:

DETAILS OF INCIDENT/ACCIDENT

NATURE & EXTENT OF INJURIES:

WHAT ACTION WAS TAKEN: – FIRST AID – AMBULANCE CALLED – HOSPITAL – POLICE – OTHER (PLEASE SPECIFY)

WITNESS(ES)

NAME:	CONTACT:
NAME:	CONTACT:

ACTIONS WHICH COULD HAVE PREVENTED THE INCIDENT

FORM COMPLETED BY:	DATE:
APPROVED BY:	POSITION:
SIGNATURE:	DATE:

INCIDENT / ACCIDENT FORM

INCIDENT DATE:	INCIDENT TIME:
LOCATION:	DATE & TIME REPORTED:

PERSON INJURED / INVOLVED: – EMPLOYEE – VISITOR – GENERAL PUBLIC – CONTRACTOR – OTHER

FULL NAME:

ADDRESS:

PHONE:	EMAIL:

DETAILS OF INCIDENT/ACCIDENT

NATURE & EXTENT OF INJURIES:

WHAT ACTION WAS TAKEN: – FIRST AID – AMBULANCE CALLED – HOSPITAL – POLICE – OTHER (PLEASE SPECIFY)

WITNESS(ES)

NAME:	CONTACT:
NAME:	CONTACT:

ACTIONS WHICH COULD HAVE PREVENTED THE INCIDENT

FORM COMPLETED BY:	DATE:
APPROVED BY:	POSITION:
SIGNATURE:	DATE:

INCIDENT / ACCIDENT FORM

INCIDENT DATE:	INCIDENT TIME:
LOCATION:	DATE & TIME REPORTED:

PERSON INJURED / INVOLVED: - EMPLOYEE - VISITOR - GENERAL PUBLIC - CONTRACTOR - OTHER

FULL NAME:

ADDRESS:

PHONE:	EMAIL:

DETAILS OF INCIDENT/ACCIDENT

NATURE & EXTENT OF INJURIES:

WHAT ACTION WAS TAKEN: - FIRST AID - AMBULANCE CALLED - HOSPITAL - POLICE - OTHER (PLEASE SPECIFY)

WITNESS(ES)

NAME:	CONTACT:
NAME:	CONTACT:

ACTIONS WHICH COULD HAVE PREVENTED THE INCIDENT

FORM COMPLETED BY:	DATE:
APPROVED BY:	POSITION:
SIGNATURE:	DATE:

INCIDENT / ACCIDENT FORM

INCIDENT DATE:	INCIDENT TIME:
LOCATION:	DATE & TIME REPORTED:

PERSON INJURED / INVOLVED: – EMPLOYEE – VISITOR – GENERAL PUBLIC – CONTRACTOR – OTHER

FULL NAME:

ADDRESS:

PHONE:	EMAIL:

DETAILS OF INCIDENT/ACCIDENT

NATURE & EXTENT OF INJURIES:

WHAT ACTION WAS TAKEN: – FIRST AID – AMBULANCE CALLED – HOSPITAL – POLICE – OTHER (PLEASE SPECIFY)

WITNESS(ES)

NAME:	CONTACT:
NAME:	CONTACT:

ACTIONS WHICH COULD HAVE PREVENTED THE INCIDENT

FORM COMPLETED BY:	DATE:
APPROVED BY:	POSITION:
SIGNATURE:	DATE:

INCIDENT / ACCIDENT FORM

INCIDENT DATE:	INCIDENT TIME:
LOCATION:	DATE & TIME REPORTED:

PERSON INJURED / INVOLVED: – EMPLOYEE – VISITOR – GENERAL PUBLIC – CONTRACTOR – OTHER

FULL NAME:

ADDRESS:

PHONE:	EMAIL:

DETAILS OF INCIDENT/ACCIDENT

NATURE & EXTENT OF INJURIES:

WHAT ACTION WAS TAKEN: – FIRST AID – AMBULANCE CALLED – HOSPITAL – POLICE – OTHER (PLEASE SPECIFY)

WITNESS(ES)

NAME:	CONTACT:
NAME:	CONTACT:

ACTIONS WHICH COULD HAVE PREVENTED THE INCIDENT

FORM COMPLETED BY:	DATE:
APPROVED BY:	POSITION:
SIGNATURE:	DATE:

INCIDENT / ACCIDENT FORM

INCIDENT DATE:	INCIDENT TIME:
LOCATION:	DATE & TIME REPORTED:

PERSON INJURED / INVOLVED: – EMPLOYEE – VISITOR – GENERAL PUBLIC – CONTRACTOR – OTHER

FULL NAME:

ADDRESS:

PHONE:	EMAIL:

DETAILS OF INCIDENT/ACCIDENT

NATURE & EXTENT OF INJURIES:

WHAT ACTION WAS TAKEN: – FIRST AID – AMBULANCE CALLED – HOSPITAL – POLICE – OTHER (PLEASE SPECIFY)

WITNESS(ES)

NAME:	CONTACT:
NAME:	CONTACT:

ACTIONS WHICH COULD HAVE PREVENTED THE INCIDENT

FORM COMPLETED BY:	DATE:
APPROVED BY:	POSITION:
SIGNATURE:	DATE:

INCIDENT / ACCIDENT FORM

INCIDENT DATE:	INCIDENT TIME:
LOCATION:	DATE & TIME REPORTED:

PERSON INJURED / INVOLVED: - EMPLOYEE - VISITOR - GENERAL PUBLIC - CONTRACTOR - OTHER

FULL NAME:

ADDRESS:

PHONE:	EMAIL:

DETAILS OF INCIDENT/ACCIDENT

NATURE & EXTENT OF INJURIES:

WHAT ACTION WAS TAKEN: - FIRST AID - AMBULANCE CALLED - HOSPITAL - POLICE - OTHER (PLEASE SPECIFY)

WITNESS(ES)

NAME:	CONTACT:
NAME:	CONTACT:

ACTIONS WHICH COULD HAVE PREVENTED THE INCIDENT

FORM COMPLETED BY:	DATE:
APPROVED BY:	POSITION:
SIGNATURE:	DATE:

INCIDENT / ACCIDENT FORM

INCIDENT DATE:	INCIDENT TIME:
LOCATION:	DATE & TIME REPORTED:

PERSON INJURED / INVOLVED: – EMPLOYEE – VISITOR – GENERAL PUBLIC – CONTRACTOR – OTHER

FULL NAME:

ADDRESS:

PHONE:	EMAIL:

DETAILS OF INCIDENT/ACCIDENT

NATURE & EXTENT OF INJURIES:

WHAT ACTION WAS TAKEN: – FIRST AID – AMBULANCE CALLED – HOSPITAL – POLICE – OTHER (PLEASE SPECIFY)

WITNESS(ES)

NAME:	CONTACT:
NAME:	CONTACT:

ACTIONS WHICH COULD HAVE PREVENTED THE INCIDENT

FORM COMPLETED BY:	DATE:
APPROVED BY:	POSITION:
SIGNATURE:	DATE:

INCIDENT / ACCIDENT FORM

INCIDENT DATE:	INCIDENT TIME:
LOCATION:	DATE & TIME REPORTED:

PERSON INJURED / INVOLVED: – EMPLOYEE – VISITOR – GENERAL PUBLIC – CONTRACTOR – OTHER

FULL NAME:

ADDRESS:

PHONE:	EMAIL:

DETAILS OF INCIDENT/ACCIDENT

NATURE & EXTENT OF INJURIES:

WHAT ACTION WAS TAKEN: – FIRST AID – AMBULANCE CALLED – HOSPITAL – POLICE – OTHER (PLEASE SPECIFY)

WITNESS(ES)

NAME:	CONTACT:
NAME:	CONTACT:

ACTIONS WHICH COULD HAVE PREVENTED THE INCIDENT

FORM COMPLETED BY:	DATE:
APPROVED BY:	POSITION:
SIGNATURE:	DATE:

INCIDENT / ACCIDENT FORM

INCIDENT DATE:	INCIDENT TIME:
LOCATION:	DATE & TIME REPORTED:

PERSON INJURED / INVOLVED: – EMPLOYEE – VISITOR – GENERAL PUBLIC – CONTRACTOR – OTHER

FULL NAME:

ADDRESS:

PHONE:	EMAIL:

DETAILS OF INCIDENT/ACCIDENT

NATURE & EXTENT OF INJURIES:

WHAT ACTION WAS TAKEN: – FIRST AID – AMBULANCE CALLED – HOSPITAL – POLICE – OTHER (PLEASE SPECIFY)

WITNESS(ES)

NAME:	CONTACT:
NAME:	CONTACT:

ACTIONS WHICH COULD HAVE PREVENTED THE INCIDENT

FORM COMPLETED BY:	DATE:
APPROVED BY:	POSITION:
SIGNATURE:	DATE:

INCIDENT / ACCIDENT FORM

INCIDENT DATE:	INCIDENT TIME:
LOCATION:	DATE & TIME REPORTED:

PERSON INJURED / INVOLVED: - EMPLOYEE - VISITOR - GENERAL PUBLIC - CONTRACTOR - OTHER

FULL NAME:

ADDRESS:

PHONE:	EMAIL:

DETAILS OF INCIDENT/ACCIDENT

NATURE & EXTENT OF INJURIES:

WHAT ACTION WAS TAKEN: - FIRST AID - AMBULANCE CALLED - HOSPITAL - POLICE - OTHER (PLEASE SPECIFY)

WITNESS(ES)

NAME:	CONTACT:
NAME:	CONTACT:

ACTIONS WHICH COULD HAVE PREVENTED THE INCIDENT

FORM COMPLETED BY:	DATE:
APPROVED BY:	POSITION:
SIGNATURE:	DATE:

INCIDENT / ACCIDENT FORM

INCIDENT DATE:	INCIDENT TIME:
LOCATION:	DATE & TIME REPORTED:

PERSON INJURED / INVOLVED: – EMPLOYEE – VISITOR – GENERAL PUBLIC – CONTRACTOR – OTHER

FULL NAME:

ADDRESS:

PHONE:	EMAIL:

DETAILS OF INCIDENT/ACCIDENT

NATURE & EXTENT OF INJURIES:

WHAT ACTION WAS TAKEN: – FIRST AID – AMBULANCE CALLED – HOSPITAL – POLICE – OTHER (PLEASE SPECIFY)

WITNESS(ES)

NAME:	CONTACT:
NAME:	CONTACT:

ACTIONS WHICH COULD HAVE PREVENTED THE INCIDENT

FORM COMPLETED BY:	DATE:
APPROVED BY:	POSITION:
SIGNATURE:	DATE:

INCIDENT / ACCIDENT FORM

INCIDENT DATE:	INCIDENT TIME:
LOCATION:	DATE & TIME REPORTED:

PERSON INJURED / INVOLVED: – EMPLOYEE – VISITOR – GENERAL PUBLIC – CONTRACTOR – OTHER

FULL NAME:

ADDRESS:

PHONE:	EMAIL:

DETAILS OF INCIDENT/ACCIDENT

NATURE & EXTENT OF INJURIES:

WHAT ACTION WAS TAKEN: – FIRST AID – AMBULANCE CALLED – HOSPITAL – POLICE – OTHER (PLEASE SPECIFY)

WITNESS(ES)

NAME:	CONTACT:
NAME:	CONTACT:

ACTIONS WHICH COULD HAVE PREVENTED THE INCIDENT

FORM COMPLETED BY:	DATE:
APPROVED BY:	POSITION:
SIGNATURE:	DATE:

INCIDENT / ACCIDENT FORM

INCIDENT DATE:	INCIDENT TIME:
LOCATION:	DATE & TIME REPORTED:

PERSON INJURED / INVOLVED: – EMPLOYEE – VISITOR – GENERAL PUBLIC – CONTRACTOR – OTHER

FULL NAME:

ADDRESS:

PHONE:	EMAIL:

DETAILS OF INCIDENT/ACCIDENT

NATURE & EXTENT OF INJURIES:

WHAT ACTION WAS TAKEN: – FIRST AID – AMBULANCE CALLED – HOSPITAL – POLICE – OTHER (PLEASE SPECIFY)

WITNESS(ES)

NAME:	CONTACT:
NAME:	CONTACT:

ACTIONS WHICH COULD HAVE PREVENTED THE INCIDENT

FORM COMPLETED BY:	DATE:
APPROVED BY:	POSITION:
SIGNATURE:	DATE:

INCIDENT / ACCIDENT FORM

INCIDENT DATE:	INCIDENT TIME:
LOCATION:	DATE & TIME REPORTED:

PERSON INJURED / INVOLVED: - EMPLOYEE - VISITOR - GENERAL PUBLIC - CONTRACTOR - OTHER

FULL NAME:

ADDRESS:

PHONE:	EMAIL:

DETAILS OF INCIDENT/ACCIDENT

NATURE & EXTENT OF INJURIES:

WHAT ACTION WAS TAKEN: - FIRST AID - AMBULANCE CALLED - HOSPITAL - POLICE - OTHER (PLEASE SPECIFY)

WITNESS(ES)

NAME:	CONTACT:
NAME:	CONTACT:

ACTIONS WHICH COULD HAVE PREVENTED THE INCIDENT

FORM COMPLETED BY:	DATE:
APPROVED BY:	POSITION:
SIGNATURE:	DATE:

INCIDENT / ACCIDENT FORM

INCIDENT DATE:	INCIDENT TIME:
LOCATION:	DATE & TIME REPORTED:

PERSON INJURED / INVOLVED: – EMPLOYEE – VISITOR – GENERAL PUBLIC – CONTRACTOR – OTHER

FULL NAME:

ADDRESS:

PHONE:	EMAIL:

DETAILS OF INCIDENT/ACCIDENT

NATURE & EXTENT OF INJURIES:

WHAT ACTION WAS TAKEN: – FIRST AID – AMBULANCE CALLED – HOSPITAL – POLICE – OTHER (PLEASE SPECIFY)

WITNESS(ES)

NAME:	CONTACT:
NAME:	CONTACT:

ACTIONS WHICH COULD HAVE PREVENTED THE INCIDENT

FORM COMPLETED BY:	DATE:
APPROVED BY:	POSITION:
SIGNATURE:	DATE:

INCIDENT / ACCIDENT FORM

INCIDENT DATE:	INCIDENT TIME:
LOCATION:	DATE & TIME REPORTED:

PERSON INJURED / INVOLVED: – EMPLOYEE – VISITOR – GENERAL PUBLIC – CONTRACTOR – OTHER

FULL NAME:

ADDRESS:

PHONE:	EMAIL:

DETAILS OF INCIDENT/ACCIDENT

NATURE & EXTENT OF INJURIES:

WHAT ACTION WAS TAKEN: – FIRST AID – AMBULANCE CALLED – HOSPITAL – POLICE – OTHER (PLEASE SPECIFY)

WITNESS(ES)

NAME:	CONTACT:
NAME:	CONTACT:

ACTIONS WHICH COULD HAVE PREVENTED THE INCIDENT

FORM COMPLETED BY:	DATE:
APPROVED BY:	POSITION:
SIGNATURE:	DATE:

INCIDENT / ACCIDENT FORM

INCIDENT DATE:	INCIDENT TIME:
LOCATION:	DATE & TIME REPORTED:

PERSON INJURED / INVOLVED: – EMPLOYEE – VISITOR – GENERAL PUBLIC – CONTRACTOR – OTHER

FULL NAME:

ADDRESS:

PHONE:	EMAIL:

DETAILS OF INCIDENT/ACCIDENT

NATURE & EXTENT OF INJURIES:

WHAT ACTION WAS TAKEN: – FIRST AID – AMBULANCE CALLED – HOSPITAL – POLICE – OTHER (PLEASE SPECIFY)

WITNESS(ES)

NAME:	CONTACT:
NAME:	CONTACT:

ACTIONS WHICH COULD HAVE PREVENTED THE INCIDENT

FORM COMPLETED BY:	DATE:
APPROVED BY:	POSITION:
SIGNATURE:	DATE:

INCIDENT / ACCIDENT FORM

INCIDENT DATE:	INCIDENT TIME:
LOCATION:	DATE & TIME REPORTED:

PERSON INJURED / INVOLVED: - EMPLOYEE - VISITOR - GENERAL PUBLIC - CONTRACTOR - OTHER

FULL NAME:

ADDRESS:

PHONE:	EMAIL:

DETAILS OF INCIDENT/ACCIDENT

NATURE & EXTENT OF INJURIES:

WHAT ACTION WAS TAKEN: - FIRST AID - AMBULANCE CALLED - HOSPITAL - POLICE - OTHER (PLEASE SPECIFY)

WITNESS(ES)

NAME:	CONTACT:
NAME:	CONTACT:

ACTIONS WHICH COULD HAVE PREVENTED THE INCIDENT

FORM COMPLETED BY:	DATE:
APPROVED BY:	POSITION:
SIGNATURE:	DATE:

INCIDENT / ACCIDENT FORM

INCIDENT DATE:	INCIDENT TIME:
LOCATION:	DATE & TIME REPORTED:

PERSON INJURED / INVOLVED: - EMPLOYEE - VISITOR - GENERAL PUBLIC - CONTRACTOR - OTHER

FULL NAME:

ADDRESS:

PHONE:	EMAIL:

DETAILS OF INCIDENT/ACCIDENT

NATURE & EXTENT OF INJURIES:

WHAT ACTION WAS TAKEN: - FIRST AID - AMBULANCE CALLED - HOSPITAL - POLICE - OTHER (PLEASE SPECIFY)

WITNESS(ES)

NAME:	CONTACT:
NAME:	CONTACT:

ACTIONS WHICH COULD HAVE PREVENTED THE INCIDENT

FORM COMPLETED BY:	DATE:
APPROVED BY:	POSITION:
SIGNATURE:	DATE:

INCIDENT / ACCIDENT FORM

INCIDENT DATE:	INCIDENT TIME:
LOCATION:	DATE & TIME REPORTED:

PERSON INJURED / INVOLVED: – EMPLOYEE – VISITOR – GENERAL PUBLIC – CONTRACTOR – OTHER

FULL NAME:

ADDRESS:

PHONE:	EMAIL:

DETAILS OF INCIDENT/ACCIDENT

NATURE & EXTENT OF INJURIES:

WHAT ACTION WAS TAKEN: – FIRST AID – AMBULANCE CALLED – HOSPITAL – POLICE – OTHER (PLEASE SPECIFY)

WITNESS(ES)

NAME:	CONTACT:
NAME:	CONTACT:

ACTIONS WHICH COULD HAVE PREVENTED THE INCIDENT

FORM COMPLETED BY:	DATE:
APPROVED BY:	POSITION:
SIGNATURE:	DATE:

INCIDENT / ACCIDENT FORM

INCIDENT DATE:	INCIDENT TIME:
LOCATION:	DATE & TIME REPORTED:

PERSON INJURED / INVOLVED: – EMPLOYEE – VISITOR – GENERAL PUBLIC – CONTRACTOR – OTHER

FULL NAME:

ADDRESS:

PHONE:	EMAIL:

DETAILS OF INCIDENT/ACCIDENT

NATURE & EXTENT OF INJURIES:

WHAT ACTION WAS TAKEN: – FIRST AID – AMBULANCE CALLED – HOSPITAL – POLICE – OTHER (PLEASE SPECIFY)

WITNESS(ES)

NAME:	CONTACT:
NAME:	CONTACT:

ACTIONS WHICH COULD HAVE PREVENTED THE INCIDENT

FORM COMPLETED BY:	DATE:
APPROVED BY:	POSITION:
SIGNATURE:	DATE:

INCIDENT / ACCIDENT FORM

INCIDENT DATE:		INCIDENT TIME:	
LOCATION:		DATE & TIME REPORTED:	

PERSON INJURED / INVOLVED: - EMPLOYEE - VISITOR - GENERAL PUBLIC - CONTRACTOR - OTHER

FULL NAME:

ADDRESS:

PHONE:		EMAIL:	

DETAILS OF INCIDENT/ACCIDENT

NATURE & EXTENT OF INJURIES:

WHAT ACTION WAS TAKEN: - FIRST AID - AMBULANCE CALLED - HOSPITAL - POLICE - OTHER (PLEASE SPECIFY)

WITNESS(ES)

NAME:		CONTACT:	
NAME:		CONTACT:	

ACTIONS WHICH COULD HAVE PREVENTED THE INCIDENT

FORM COMPLETED BY:		DATE:	
APPROVED BY:		POSITION:	
SIGNATURE:		DATE:	

INCIDENT / ACCIDENT FORM

INCIDENT DATE:	INCIDENT TIME:
LOCATION:	DATE & TIME REPORTED:

PERSON INJURED / INVOLVED: – EMPLOYEE – VISITOR – GENERAL PUBLIC – CONTRACTOR – OTHER

FULL NAME:

ADDRESS:

PHONE:	EMAIL:

DETAILS OF INCIDENT/ACCIDENT

NATURE & EXTENT OF INJURIES:

WHAT ACTION WAS TAKEN: – FIRST AID – AMBULANCE CALLED – HOSPITAL – POLICE – OTHER (PLEASE SPECIFY)

WITNESS(ES)

NAME:	CONTACT:
NAME:	CONTACT:

ACTIONS WHICH COULD HAVE PREVENTED THE INCIDENT

FORM COMPLETED BY:	DATE:
APPROVED BY:	POSITION:
SIGNATURE:	DATE:

INCIDENT / ACCIDENT FORM

INCIDENT DATE:	INCIDENT TIME:
LOCATION:	DATE & TIME REPORTED:

PERSON INJURED / INVOLVED: – EMPLOYEE – VISITOR – GENERAL PUBLIC – CONTRACTOR – OTHER

FULL NAME:

ADDRESS:

PHONE:	EMAIL:

DETAILS OF INCIDENT/ACCIDENT

NATURE & EXTENT OF INJURIES:

WHAT ACTION WAS TAKEN: – FIRST AID – AMBULANCE CALLED – HOSPITAL – POLICE – OTHER (PLEASE SPECIFY)

WITNESS(ES)

NAME:	CONTACT:
NAME:	CONTACT:

ACTIONS WHICH COULD HAVE PREVENTED THE INCIDENT

FORM COMPLETED BY:	DATE:
APPROVED BY:	POSITION:
SIGNATURE:	DATE:

INCIDENT / ACCIDENT FORM

INCIDENT DATE:	INCIDENT TIME:
LOCATION:	DATE & TIME REPORTED:

PERSON INJURED / INVOLVED: – EMPLOYEE – VISITOR – GENERAL PUBLIC – CONTRACTOR – OTHER

FULL NAME:

ADDRESS:

PHONE:	EMAIL:

DETAILS OF INCIDENT/ACCIDENT

NATURE & EXTENT OF INJURIES:

WHAT ACTION WAS TAKEN: – FIRST AID – AMBULANCE CALLED – HOSPITAL – POLICE – OTHER (PLEASE SPECIFY)

WITNESS(ES)

NAME:	CONTACT:
NAME:	CONTACT:

ACTIONS WHICH COULD HAVE PREVENTED THE INCIDENT

FORM COMPLETED BY:	DATE:
APPROVED BY:	POSITION:
SIGNATURE:	DATE:

INCIDENT / ACCIDENT FORM

INCIDENT DATE:	INCIDENT TIME:
LOCATION:	DATE & TIME REPORTED:

PERSON INJURED / INVOLVED: - EMPLOYEE - VISITOR - GENERAL PUBLIC - CONTRACTOR - OTHER

FULL NAME:

ADDRESS:

PHONE:	EMAIL:

DETAILS OF INCIDENT/ACCIDENT

NATURE & EXTENT OF INJURIES:

WHAT ACTION WAS TAKEN: - FIRST AID - AMBULANCE CALLED - HOSPITAL - POLICE - OTHER (PLEASE SPECIFY)

WITNESS(ES)

NAME:	CONTACT:
NAME:	CONTACT:

ACTIONS WHICH COULD HAVE PREVENTED THE INCIDENT

FORM COMPLETED BY:	DATE:
APPROVED BY:	POSITION:
SIGNATURE:	DATE:

INCIDENT / ACCIDENT FORM

INCIDENT DATE:	INCIDENT TIME:
LOCATION:	DATE & TIME REPORTED:

PERSON INJURED / INVOLVED: – EMPLOYEE – VISITOR – GENERAL PUBLIC – CONTRACTOR – OTHER

FULL NAME:

ADDRESS:

PHONE:	EMAIL:

DETAILS OF INCIDENT/ACCIDENT

NATURE & EXTENT OF INJURIES:

WHAT ACTION WAS TAKEN: – FIRST AID – AMBULANCE CALLED – HOSPITAL – POLICE – OTHER (PLEASE SPECIFY)

WITNESS(ES)

NAME:	CONTACT:
NAME:	CONTACT:

ACTIONS WHICH COULD HAVE PREVENTED THE INCIDENT

FORM COMPLETED BY:	DATE:
APPROVED BY:	POSITION:
SIGNATURE:	DATE:

INCIDENT / ACCIDENT FORM

INCIDENT DATE:	INCIDENT TIME:
LOCATION:	DATE & TIME REPORTED:

PERSON INJURED / INVOLVED: - EMPLOYEE - VISITOR - GENERAL PUBLIC - CONTRACTOR - OTHER

FULL NAME:

ADDRESS:

PHONE:	EMAIL:

DETAILS OF INCIDENT/ACCIDENT

NATURE & EXTENT OF INJURIES:

WHAT ACTION WAS TAKEN: - FIRST AID - AMBULANCE CALLED - HOSPITAL - POLICE - OTHER (PLEASE SPECIFY)

WITNESS(ES)

NAME:	CONTACT:
NAME:	CONTACT:

ACTIONS WHICH COULD HAVE PREVENTED THE INCIDENT

FORM COMPLETED BY:	DATE:
APPROVED BY:	POSITION:
SIGNATURE:	DATE:

INCIDENT / ACCIDENT FORM

INCIDENT DATE:	INCIDENT TIME:
LOCATION:	DATE & TIME REPORTED:

PERSON INJURED / INVOLVED: - EMPLOYEE - VISITOR - GENERAL PUBLIC - CONTRACTOR - OTHER

FULL NAME:

ADDRESS:

PHONE:	EMAIL:

DETAILS OF INCIDENT/ACCIDENT

NATURE & EXTENT OF INJURIES:

WHAT ACTION WAS TAKEN: - FIRST AID - AMBULANCE CALLED - HOSPITAL - POLICE - OTHER (PLEASE SPECIFY)

WITNESS(ES)

NAME:	CONTACT:
NAME:	CONTACT:

ACTIONS WHICH COULD HAVE PREVENTED THE INCIDENT

FORM COMPLETED BY:	DATE:
APPROVED BY:	POSITION:
SIGNATURE:	DATE:

INCIDENT / ACCIDENT FORM

INCIDENT DATE:	INCIDENT TIME:
LOCATION:	DATE & TIME REPORTED:

PERSON INJURED / INVOLVED: – EMPLOYEE – VISITOR – GENERAL PUBLIC – CONTRACTOR – OTHER

FULL NAME:

ADDRESS:

PHONE:	EMAIL:

DETAILS OF INCIDENT/ACCIDENT

NATURE & EXTENT OF INJURIES:

WHAT ACTION WAS TAKEN: – FIRST AID – AMBULANCE CALLED – HOSPITAL – POLICE – OTHER (PLEASE SPECIFY)

WITNESS(ES)

NAME:	CONTACT:
NAME:	CONTACT:

ACTIONS WHICH COULD HAVE PREVENTED THE INCIDENT

FORM COMPLETED BY:	DATE:
APPROVED BY:	POSITION:
SIGNATURE:	DATE:

INCIDENT / ACCIDENT FORM

INCIDENT DATE:	INCIDENT TIME:
LOCATION:	DATE & TIME REPORTED:

PERSON INJURED / INVOLVED: – EMPLOYEE – VISITOR – GENERAL PUBLIC – CONTRACTOR – OTHER

FULL NAME:

ADDRESS:

PHONE:	EMAIL:

DETAILS OF INCIDENT/ACCIDENT

NATURE & EXTENT OF INJURIES:

WHAT ACTION WAS TAKEN: – FIRST AID – AMBULANCE CALLED – HOSPITAL – POLICE – OTHER (PLEASE SPECIFY)

WITNESS(ES)

NAME:	CONTACT:
NAME:	CONTACT:

ACTIONS WHICH COULD HAVE PREVENTED THE INCIDENT

FORM COMPLETED BY:	DATE:
APPROVED BY:	POSITION:
SIGNATURE:	DATE:

INCIDENT / ACCIDENT FORM

INCIDENT DATE:	INCIDENT TIME:
LOCATION:	DATE & TIME REPORTED:

PERSON INJURED / INVOLVED: – EMPLOYEE – VISITOR – GENERAL PUBLIC – CONTRACTOR – OTHER

FULL NAME:

ADDRESS:

PHONE:	EMAIL:

DETAILS OF INCIDENT/ACCIDENT

NATURE & EXTENT OF INJURIES:

WHAT ACTION WAS TAKEN: – FIRST AID – AMBULANCE CALLED – HOSPITAL – POLICE – OTHER (PLEASE SPECIFY)

WITNESS(ES)

NAME:	CONTACT:
NAME:	CONTACT:

ACTIONS WHICH COULD HAVE PREVENTED THE INCIDENT

FORM COMPLETED BY:	DATE:
APPROVED BY:	POSITION:
SIGNATURE:	DATE:

INCIDENT / ACCIDENT FORM

INCIDENT DATE:	INCIDENT TIME:
LOCATION:	DATE & TIME REPORTED:

PERSON INJURED / INVOLVED: – EMPLOYEE – VISITOR – GENERAL PUBLIC – CONTRACTOR – OTHER

FULL NAME:

ADDRESS:

PHONE:	EMAIL:

DETAILS OF INCIDENT/ACCIDENT

NATURE & EXTENT OF INJURIES:

WHAT ACTION WAS TAKEN: – FIRST AID – AMBULANCE CALLED – HOSPITAL – POLICE – OTHER (PLEASE SPECIFY)

WITNESS(ES)

NAME:	CONTACT:
NAME:	CONTACT:

ACTIONS WHICH COULD HAVE PREVENTED THE INCIDENT

FORM COMPLETED BY:	DATE:
APPROVED BY:	POSITION:
SIGNATURE:	DATE:

INCIDENT / ACCIDENT FORM

INCIDENT DATE:	INCIDENT TIME:
LOCATION:	DATE & TIME REPORTED:

PERSON INJURED / INVOLVED: - EMPLOYEE - VISITOR - GENERAL PUBLIC - CONTRACTOR - OTHER

FULL NAME:

ADDRESS:

PHONE:	EMAIL:

DETAILS OF INCIDENT/ACCIDENT

NATURE & EXTENT OF INJURIES:

WHAT ACTION WAS TAKEN: - FIRST AID - AMBULANCE CALLED - HOSPITAL - POLICE - OTHER (PLEASE SPECIFY)

WITNESS(ES)

NAME:	CONTACT:
NAME:	CONTACT:

ACTIONS WHICH COULD HAVE PREVENTED THE INCIDENT

FORM COMPLETED BY:	DATE:
APPROVED BY:	POSITION:
SIGNATURE:	DATE:

INCIDENT / ACCIDENT FORM

INCIDENT DATE:	INCIDENT TIME:
LOCATION:	DATE & TIME REPORTED:

PERSON INJURED / INVOLVED: – EMPLOYEE – VISITOR – GENERAL PUBLIC – CONTRACTOR – OTHER

FULL NAME:

ADDRESS:

PHONE:	EMAIL:

DETAILS OF INCIDENT/ACCIDENT

NATURE & EXTENT OF INJURIES:

WHAT ACTION WAS TAKEN: – FIRST AID – AMBULANCE CALLED – HOSPITAL – POLICE – OTHER (PLEASE SPECIFY)

WITNESS(ES)

NAME:	CONTACT:
NAME:	CONTACT:

ACTIONS WHICH COULD HAVE PREVENTED THE INCIDENT

FORM COMPLETED BY:	DATE:
APPROVED BY:	POSITION:
SIGNATURE:	DATE:

INCIDENT / ACCIDENT FORM

INCIDENT DATE:	INCIDENT TIME:
LOCATION:	DATE & TIME REPORTED:

PERSON INJURED / INVOLVED: – EMPLOYEE – VISITOR – GENERAL PUBLIC – CONTRACTOR – OTHER

FULL NAME:

ADDRESS:

PHONE:	EMAIL:

DETAILS OF INCIDENT/ACCIDENT

NATURE & EXTENT OF INJURIES:

WHAT ACTION WAS TAKEN: – FIRST AID – AMBULANCE CALLED – HOSPITAL – POLICE – OTHER (PLEASE SPECIFY)

WITNESS(ES)

NAME:	CONTACT:
NAME:	CONTACT:

ACTIONS WHICH COULD HAVE PREVENTED THE INCIDENT

FORM COMPLETED BY:	DATE:
APPROVED BY:	POSITION:
SIGNATURE:	DATE:

INCIDENT / ACCIDENT FORM

INCIDENT DATE:	INCIDENT TIME:
LOCATION:	DATE & TIME REPORTED:

PERSON INJURED / INVOLVED: - EMPLOYEE - VISITOR - GENERAL PUBLIC - CONTRACTOR - OTHER

FULL NAME:

ADDRESS:

PHONE:	EMAIL:

DETAILS OF INCIDENT/ACCIDENT

NATURE & EXTENT OF INJURIES:

WHAT ACTION WAS TAKEN: - FIRST AID - AMBULANCE CALLED - HOSPITAL - POLICE - OTHER (PLEASE SPECIFY)

WITNESS(ES)

NAME:	CONTACT:
NAME:	CONTACT:

ACTIONS WHICH COULD HAVE PREVENTED THE INCIDENT

FORM COMPLETED BY:	DATE:
APPROVED BY:	POSITION:
SIGNATURE:	DATE:

INCIDENT / ACCIDENT FORM

INCIDENT DATE:	INCIDENT TIME:
LOCATION:	DATE & TIME REPORTED:

PERSON INJURED / INVOLVED: - EMPLOYEE - VISITOR - GENERAL PUBLIC - CONTRACTOR - OTHER

FULL NAME:

ADDRESS:

PHONE:	EMAIL:

DETAILS OF INCIDENT/ACCIDENT

NATURE & EXTENT OF INJURIES:

WHAT ACTION WAS TAKEN: - FIRST AID - AMBULANCE CALLED - HOSPITAL - POLICE - OTHER (PLEASE SPECIFY)

WITNESS(ES)

NAME:	CONTACT:
NAME:	CONTACT:

ACTIONS WHICH COULD HAVE PREVENTED THE INCIDENT

FORM COMPLETED BY:	DATE:
APPROVED BY:	POSITION:
SIGNATURE:	DATE:

INCIDENT / ACCIDENT FORM

INCIDENT DATE:	INCIDENT TIME:
LOCATION:	DATE & TIME REPORTED:

PERSON INJURED / INVOLVED: - EMPLOYEE - VISITOR - GENERAL PUBLIC - CONTRACTOR - OTHER

FULL NAME:

ADDRESS:

PHONE:	EMAIL:

DETAILS OF INCIDENT/ACCIDENT

NATURE & EXTENT OF INJURIES:

WHAT ACTION WAS TAKEN: - FIRST AID - AMBULANCE CALLED - HOSPITAL - POLICE - OTHER (PLEASE SPECIFY)

WITNESS(ES)

NAME:	CONTACT:
NAME:	CONTACT:

ACTIONS WHICH COULD HAVE PREVENTED THE INCIDENT

FORM COMPLETED BY:	DATE:
APPROVED BY:	POSITION:
SIGNATURE:	DATE:

INCIDENT / ACCIDENT FORM

INCIDENT DATE:	INCIDENT TIME:
LOCATION:	DATE & TIME REPORTED:

PERSON INJURED / INVOLVED: – EMPLOYEE – VISITOR – GENERAL PUBLIC – CONTRACTOR – OTHER

FULL NAME:

ADDRESS:

PHONE:	EMAIL:

DETAILS OF INCIDENT/ACCIDENT

NATURE & EXTENT OF INJURIES:

WHAT ACTION WAS TAKEN: – FIRST AID – AMBULANCE CALLED – HOSPITAL – POLICE – OTHER (PLEASE SPECIFY)

WITNESS(ES)

NAME:	CONTACT:
NAME:	CONTACT:

ACTIONS WHICH COULD HAVE PREVENTED THE INCIDENT

FORM COMPLETED BY:	DATE:
APPROVED BY:	POSITION:
SIGNATURE:	DATE:

INCIDENT / ACCIDENT FORM

INCIDENT DATE:	INCIDENT TIME:
LOCATION:	DATE & TIME REPORTED:

PERSON INJURED / INVOLVED: - EMPLOYEE - VISITOR - GENERAL PUBLIC - CONTRACTOR - OTHER

FULL NAME:

ADDRESS:

PHONE:	EMAIL:

DETAILS OF INCIDENT/ACCIDENT

NATURE & EXTENT OF INJURIES:

WHAT ACTION WAS TAKEN: - FIRST AID - AMBULANCE CALLED - HOSPITAL - POLICE - OTHER (PLEASE SPECIFY)

WITNESS(ES)

NAME:	CONTACT:
NAME:	CONTACT:

ACTIONS WHICH COULD HAVE PREVENTED THE INCIDENT

FORM COMPLETED BY:	DATE:
APPROVED BY:	POSITION:
SIGNATURE:	DATE:

INCIDENT / ACCIDENT FORM

INCIDENT DATE:	INCIDENT TIME:
LOCATION:	DATE & TIME REPORTED:

PERSON INJURED / INVOLVED: - EMPLOYEE - VISITOR - GENERAL PUBLIC - CONTRACTOR - OTHER

FULL NAME:

ADDRESS:

PHONE:	EMAIL:

DETAILS OF INCIDENT/ACCIDENT

NATURE & EXTENT OF INJURIES:

WHAT ACTION WAS TAKEN: - FIRST AID - AMBULANCE CALLED - HOSPITAL - POLICE - OTHER (PLEASE SPECIFY)

WITNESS(ES)

NAME:	CONTACT:
NAME:	CONTACT:

ACTIONS WHICH COULD HAVE PREVENTED THE INCIDENT

FORM COMPLETED BY:	DATE:
APPROVED BY:	POSITION:
SIGNATURE:	DATE:

INCIDENT / ACCIDENT FORM

INCIDENT DATE: | INCIDENT TIME:

LOCATION: | DATE & TIME REPORTED:

PERSON INJURED / INVOLVED: – EMPLOYEE – VISITOR – GENERAL PUBLIC – CONTRACTOR – OTHER

FULL NAME:

ADDRESS:

PHONE: | EMAIL:

DETAILS OF INCIDENT/ACCIDENT

NATURE & EXTENT OF INJURIES:

WHAT ACTION WAS TAKEN: – FIRST AID – AMBULANCE CALLED – HOSPITAL – POLICE – OTHER (PLEASE SPECIFY)

WITNESS(ES)

NAME: | CONTACT:

NAME: | CONTACT:

ACTIONS WHICH COULD HAVE PREVENTED THE INCIDENT

FORM COMPLETED BY: | DATE:

APPROVED BY: | POSITION:

SIGNATURE: | DATE:

INCIDENT / ACCIDENT FORM

INCIDENT DATE:	INCIDENT TIME:
LOCATION:	DATE & TIME REPORTED:

PERSON INJURED / INVOLVED: – EMPLOYEE – VISITOR – GENERAL PUBLIC – CONTRACTOR – OTHER

FULL NAME:

ADDRESS:

PHONE:	EMAIL:

DETAILS OF INCIDENT/ACCIDENT

NATURE & EXTENT OF INJURIES:

WHAT ACTION WAS TAKEN: – FIRST AID – AMBULANCE CALLED – HOSPITAL – POLICE – OTHER (PLEASE SPECIFY)

WITNESS(ES)

NAME:	CONTACT:
NAME:	CONTACT:

ACTIONS WHICH COULD HAVE PREVENTED THE INCIDENT

FORM COMPLETED BY:	DATE:
APPROVED BY:	POSITION:
SIGNATURE:	DATE:

INCIDENT / ACCIDENT FORM

INCIDENT DATE:	INCIDENT TIME:
LOCATION:	DATE & TIME REPORTED:

PERSON INJURED / INVOLVED: - EMPLOYEE - VISITOR - GENERAL PUBLIC - CONTRACTOR - OTHER

FULL NAME:

ADDRESS:

PHONE:	EMAIL:

DETAILS OF INCIDENT/ACCIDENT

NATURE & EXTENT OF INJURIES:

WHAT ACTION WAS TAKEN: - FIRST AID - AMBULANCE CALLED - HOSPITAL - POLICE - OTHER (PLEASE SPECIFY)

WITNESS(ES)

NAME:	CONTACT:
NAME:	CONTACT:

ACTIONS WHICH COULD HAVE PREVENTED THE INCIDENT

FORM COMPLETED BY:	DATE:
APPROVED BY:	POSITION:
SIGNATURE:	DATE:

INCIDENT / ACCIDENT FORM

INCIDENT DATE:	INCIDENT TIME:
LOCATION:	DATE & TIME REPORTED:

PERSON INJURED / INVOLVED: - EMPLOYEE - VISITOR - GENERAL PUBLIC - CONTRACTOR - OTHER

FULL NAME:

ADDRESS:

PHONE:	EMAIL:

DETAILS OF INCIDENT/ACCIDENT

NATURE & EXTENT OF INJURIES:

WHAT ACTION WAS TAKEN: - FIRST AID - AMBULANCE CALLED - HOSPITAL - POLICE - OTHER (PLEASE SPECIFY)

WITNESS(ES)

NAME:	CONTACT:
NAME:	CONTACT:

ACTIONS WHICH COULD HAVE PREVENTED THE INCIDENT

FORM COMPLETED BY:	DATE:
APPROVED BY:	POSITION:
SIGNATURE:	DATE:

INCIDENT / ACCIDENT FORM

INCIDENT DATE:	INCIDENT TIME:
LOCATION:	DATE & TIME REPORTED:

PERSON INJURED / INVOLVED: - EMPLOYEE - VISITOR - GENERAL PUBLIC - CONTRACTOR - OTHER

FULL NAME:

ADDRESS:

PHONE:	EMAIL:

DETAILS OF INCIDENT/ACCIDENT

NATURE & EXTENT OF INJURIES:

WHAT ACTION WAS TAKEN: - FIRST AID - AMBULANCE CALLED - HOSPITAL - POLICE - OTHER (PLEASE SPECIFY)

WITNESS(ES)

NAME:	CONTACT:
NAME:	CONTACT:

ACTIONS WHICH COULD HAVE PREVENTED THE INCIDENT

FORM COMPLETED BY:	DATE:
APPROVED BY:	POSITION:
SIGNATURE:	DATE:

INCIDENT / ACCIDENT FORM

INCIDENT DATE:	INCIDENT TIME:
LOCATION:	DATE & TIME REPORTED:

PERSON INJURED / INVOLVED: – EMPLOYEE – VISITOR – GENERAL PUBLIC – CONTRACTOR – OTHER

FULL NAME:

ADDRESS:

PHONE:	EMAIL:

DETAILS OF INCIDENT/ACCIDENT

NATURE & EXTENT OF INJURIES:

WHAT ACTION WAS TAKEN: – FIRST AID – AMBULANCE CALLED – HOSPITAL – POLICE – OTHER (PLEASE SPECIFY)

WITNESS(ES)

NAME:	CONTACT:
NAME:	CONTACT:

ACTIONS WHICH COULD HAVE PREVENTED THE INCIDENT

FORM COMPLETED BY:	DATE:
APPROVED BY:	POSITION:
SIGNATURE:	DATE:

INCIDENT / ACCIDENT FORM

INCIDENT DATE:	INCIDENT TIME:
LOCATION:	DATE & TIME REPORTED:

PERSON INJURED / INVOLVED: – EMPLOYEE – VISITOR – GENERAL PUBLIC – CONTRACTOR – OTHER

FULL NAME:

ADDRESS:

PHONE:	EMAIL:

DETAILS OF INCIDENT/ACCIDENT

NATURE & EXTENT OF INJURIES:

WHAT ACTION WAS TAKEN: – FIRST AID – AMBULANCE CALLED – HOSPITAL – POLICE – OTHER (PLEASE SPECIFY)

WITNESS(ES)

NAME:	CONTACT:
NAME:	CONTACT:

ACTIONS WHICH COULD HAVE PREVENTED THE INCIDENT

FORM COMPLETED BY:	DATE:
APPROVED BY:	POSITION:
SIGNATURE:	DATE:

INCIDENT / ACCIDENT FORM

INCIDENT DATE:	INCIDENT TIME:
LOCATION:	DATE & TIME REPORTED:

PERSON INJURED / INVOLVED: - EMPLOYEE - VISITOR - GENERAL PUBLIC - CONTRACTOR - OTHER

FULL NAME:

ADDRESS:

PHONE:	EMAIL:

DETAILS OF INCIDENT/ACCIDENT

NATURE & EXTENT OF INJURIES:

WHAT ACTION WAS TAKEN: - FIRST AID - AMBULANCE CALLED - HOSPITAL - POLICE - OTHER (PLEASE SPECIFY)

WITNESS(ES)

NAME:	CONTACT:
NAME:	CONTACT:

ACTIONS WHICH COULD HAVE PREVENTED THE INCIDENT

FORM COMPLETED BY:	DATE:
APPROVED BY:	POSITION:
SIGNATURE:	DATE:

INCIDENT / ACCIDENT FORM

INCIDENT DATE:	INCIDENT TIME:
LOCATION:	DATE & TIME REPORTED:

PERSON INJURED / INVOLVED: – EMPLOYEE – VISITOR – GENERAL PUBLIC – CONTRACTOR – OTHER

FULL NAME:

ADDRESS:

PHONE:	EMAIL:

DETAILS OF INCIDENT/ACCIDENT

NATURE & EXTENT OF INJURIES:

WHAT ACTION WAS TAKEN: – FIRST AID – AMBULANCE CALLED – HOSPITAL – POLICE – OTHER (PLEASE SPECIFY)

WITNESS(ES)

NAME:	CONTACT:
NAME:	CONTACT:

ACTIONS WHICH COULD HAVE PREVENTED THE INCIDENT

FORM COMPLETED BY:	DATE:
APPROVED BY:	POSITION:
SIGNATURE:	DATE:

INCIDENT / ACCIDENT FORM

INCIDENT DATE:	INCIDENT TIME:
LOCATION:	DATE & TIME REPORTED:

PERSON INJURED / INVOLVED: – EMPLOYEE – VISITOR – GENERAL PUBLIC – CONTRACTOR – OTHER

FULL NAME:

ADDRESS:

PHONE:	EMAIL:

DETAILS OF INCIDENT/ACCIDENT

NATURE & EXTENT OF INJURIES:

WHAT ACTION WAS TAKEN: – FIRST AID – AMBULANCE CALLED – HOSPITAL – POLICE – OTHER (PLEASE SPECIFY)

WITNESS(ES)

NAME:	CONTACT:
NAME:	CONTACT:

ACTIONS WHICH COULD HAVE PREVENTED THE INCIDENT

FORM COMPLETED BY:	DATE:
APPROVED BY:	POSITION:
SIGNATURE:	DATE:

INCIDENT / ACCIDENT FORM

INCIDENT DATE:	INCIDENT TIME:
LOCATION:	DATE & TIME REPORTED:

PERSON INJURED / INVOLVED: – EMPLOYEE – VISITOR – GENERAL PUBLIC – CONTRACTOR – OTHER

FULL NAME:

ADDRESS:

PHONE:	EMAIL:

DETAILS OF INCIDENT/ACCIDENT

NATURE & EXTENT OF INJURIES:

WHAT ACTION WAS TAKEN: – FIRST AID – AMBULANCE CALLED – HOSPITAL – POLICE – OTHER (PLEASE SPECIFY)

WITNESS(ES)

NAME:	CONTACT:
NAME:	CONTACT:

ACTIONS WHICH COULD HAVE PREVENTED THE INCIDENT

FORM COMPLETED BY:	DATE:
APPROVED BY:	POSITION:
SIGNATURE:	DATE:

INCIDENT / ACCIDENT FORM

INCIDENT DATE:	INCIDENT TIME:
LOCATION:	DATE & TIME REPORTED:

PERSON INJURED / INVOLVED: - EMPLOYEE - VISITOR - GENERAL PUBLIC - CONTRACTOR - OTHER

FULL NAME:

ADDRESS:

PHONE:	EMAIL:

DETAILS OF INCIDENT/ACCIDENT

NATURE & EXTENT OF INJURIES:

WHAT ACTION WAS TAKEN: - FIRST AID - AMBULANCE CALLED - HOSPITAL - POLICE - OTHER (PLEASE SPECIFY)

WITNESS(ES)

NAME:	CONTACT:
NAME:	CONTACT:

ACTIONS WHICH COULD HAVE PREVENTED THE INCIDENT

FORM COMPLETED BY:	DATE:
APPROVED BY:	POSITION:
SIGNATURE:	DATE:

INCIDENT / ACCIDENT FORM

INCIDENT DATE:	INCIDENT TIME:
LOCATION:	DATE & TIME REPORTED:

PERSON INJURED / INVOLVED: – EMPLOYEE – VISITOR – GENERAL PUBLIC – CONTRACTOR – OTHER

FULL NAME:

ADDRESS:

PHONE:	EMAIL:

DETAILS OF INCIDENT/ACCIDENT

NATURE & EXTENT OF INJURIES:

WHAT ACTION WAS TAKEN: – FIRST AID – AMBULANCE CALLED – HOSPITAL – POLICE – OTHER (PLEASE SPECIFY)

WITNESS(ES)

NAME:	CONTACT:
NAME:	CONTACT:

ACTIONS WHICH COULD HAVE PREVENTED THE INCIDENT

FORM COMPLETED BY:	DATE:
APPROVED BY:	POSITION:
SIGNATURE:	DATE:

INCIDENT / ACCIDENT FORM

INCIDENT DATE:	INCIDENT TIME:
LOCATION:	DATE & TIME REPORTED:

PERSON INJURED / INVOLVED: – EMPLOYEE – VISITOR – GENERAL PUBLIC – CONTRACTOR – OTHER

FULL NAME:

ADDRESS:

PHONE:	EMAIL:

DETAILS OF INCIDENT/ACCIDENT

NATURE & EXTENT OF INJURIES:

WHAT ACTION WAS TAKEN: – FIRST AID – AMBULANCE CALLED – HOSPITAL – POLICE – OTHER (PLEASE SPECIFY)

WITNESS(ES)

NAME:	CONTACT:
NAME:	CONTACT:

ACTIONS WHICH COULD HAVE PREVENTED THE INCIDENT

FORM COMPLETED BY:	DATE:
APPROVED BY:	POSITION:
SIGNATURE:	DATE:

INCIDENT / ACCIDENT FORM

INCIDENT DATE:	INCIDENT TIME:
LOCATION:	DATE & TIME REPORTED:

PERSON INJURED / INVOLVED: - EMPLOYEE - VISITOR - GENERAL PUBLIC - CONTRACTOR - OTHER

FULL NAME:

ADDRESS:

PHONE:	EMAIL:

DETAILS OF INCIDENT/ACCIDENT

NATURE & EXTENT OF INJURIES:

WHAT ACTION WAS TAKEN: - FIRST AID - AMBULANCE CALLED - HOSPITAL - POLICE - OTHER (PLEASE SPECIFY)

WITNESS(ES)

NAME:	CONTACT:
NAME:	CONTACT:

ACTIONS WHICH COULD HAVE PREVENTED THE INCIDENT

FORM COMPLETED BY:	DATE:
APPROVED BY:	POSITION:
SIGNATURE:	DATE:

INCIDENT / ACCIDENT FORM

INCIDENT DATE:	INCIDENT TIME:
LOCATION:	DATE & TIME REPORTED:

PERSON INJURED / INVOLVED: - EMPLOYEE - VISITOR - GENERAL PUBLIC - CONTRACTOR - OTHER

FULL NAME:

ADDRESS:

PHONE:	EMAIL:

DETAILS OF INCIDENT/ACCIDENT

NATURE & EXTENT OF INJURIES:

WHAT ACTION WAS TAKEN: - FIRST AID - AMBULANCE CALLED - HOSPITAL - POLICE - OTHER (PLEASE SPECIFY)

WITNESS(ES)

NAME:	CONTACT:
NAME:	CONTACT:

ACTIONS WHICH COULD HAVE PREVENTED THE INCIDENT

FORM COMPLETED BY:	DATE:
APPROVED BY:	POSITION:
SIGNATURE:	DATE:

INCIDENT / ACCIDENT FORM

INCIDENT DATE:	INCIDENT TIME:
LOCATION:	DATE & TIME REPORTED:

PERSON INJURED / INVOLVED: – EMPLOYEE – VISITOR – GENERAL PUBLIC – CONTRACTOR – OTHER

FULL NAME:

ADDRESS:

PHONE:	EMAIL:

DETAILS OF INCIDENT/ACCIDENT

NATURE & EXTENT OF INJURIES:

WHAT ACTION WAS TAKEN: – FIRST AID – AMBULANCE CALLED – HOSPITAL – POLICE – OTHER (PLEASE SPECIFY)

WITNESS(ES)

NAME:	CONTACT:
NAME:	CONTACT:

ACTIONS WHICH COULD HAVE PREVENTED THE INCIDENT

FORM COMPLETED BY:	DATE:
APPROVED BY:	POSITION:
SIGNATURE:	DATE:

INCIDENT / ACCIDENT FORM

INCIDENT DATE:	INCIDENT TIME:
LOCATION:	DATE & TIME REPORTED:

PERSON INJURED / INVOLVED: – EMPLOYEE – VISITOR – GENERAL PUBLIC – CONTRACTOR – OTHER

FULL NAME:

ADDRESS:

PHONE:	EMAIL:

DETAILS OF INCIDENT/ACCIDENT

NATURE & EXTENT OF INJURIES:

WHAT ACTION WAS TAKEN: – FIRST AID – AMBULANCE CALLED – HOSPITAL – POLICE – OTHER (PLEASE SPECIFY)

WITNESS(ES)

NAME:	CONTACT:
NAME:	CONTACT:

ACTIONS WHICH COULD HAVE PREVENTED THE INCIDENT

FORM COMPLETED BY:	DATE:
APPROVED BY:	POSITION:
SIGNATURE:	DATE:

INCIDENT / ACCIDENT FORM

INCIDENT DATE:	INCIDENT TIME:
LOCATION:	DATE & TIME REPORTED:

PERSON INJURED / INVOLVED: - EMPLOYEE - VISITOR - GENERAL PUBLIC - CONTRACTOR - OTHER

FULL NAME:

ADDRESS:

PHONE:	EMAIL:

DETAILS OF INCIDENT/ACCIDENT

NATURE & EXTENT OF INJURIES:

WHAT ACTION WAS TAKEN: - FIRST AID - AMBULANCE CALLED - HOSPITAL - POLICE - OTHER (PLEASE SPECIFY)

WITNESS(ES)

NAME:	CONTACT:
NAME:	CONTACT:

ACTIONS WHICH COULD HAVE PREVENTED THE INCIDENT

FORM COMPLETED BY:	DATE:
APPROVED BY:	POSITION:
SIGNATURE:	DATE:

INCIDENT / ACCIDENT FORM

INCIDENT DATE:	INCIDENT TIME:
LOCATION:	DATE & TIME REPORTED:

PERSON INJURED / INVOLVED: – EMPLOYEE – VISITOR – GENERAL PUBLIC – CONTRACTOR – OTHER

FULL NAME:

ADDRESS:

PHONE:	EMAIL:

DETAILS OF INCIDENT/ACCIDENT

NATURE & EXTENT OF INJURIES:

WHAT ACTION WAS TAKEN: – FIRST AID – AMBULANCE CALLED – HOSPITAL – POLICE – OTHER (PLEASE SPECIFY)

WITNESS(ES)

NAME:	CONTACT:
NAME:	CONTACT:

ACTIONS WHICH COULD HAVE PREVENTED THE INCIDENT

FORM COMPLETED BY:	DATE:
APPROVED BY:	POSITION:
SIGNATURE:	DATE:

INCIDENT / ACCIDENT FORM

INCIDENT DATE:	INCIDENT TIME:
LOCATION:	DATE & TIME REPORTED:

PERSON INJURED / INVOLVED: – EMPLOYEE – VISITOR – GENERAL PUBLIC – CONTRACTOR – OTHER

FULL NAME:

ADDRESS:

PHONE:	EMAIL:

DETAILS OF INCIDENT/ACCIDENT

NATURE & EXTENT OF INJURIES:

WHAT ACTION WAS TAKEN: – FIRST AID – AMBULANCE CALLED – HOSPITAL – POLICE – OTHER (PLEASE SPECIFY)

WITNESS(ES)

NAME:	CONTACT:
NAME:	CONTACT:

ACTIONS WHICH COULD HAVE PREVENTED THE INCIDENT

FORM COMPLETED BY:	DATE:
APPROVED BY:	POSITION:
SIGNATURE:	DATE:

INCIDENT / ACCIDENT FORM

INCIDENT DATE:	INCIDENT TIME:
LOCATION:	DATE & TIME REPORTED:

PERSON INJURED / INVOLVED: – EMPLOYEE – VISITOR – GENERAL PUBLIC – CONTRACTOR – OTHER

FULL NAME:

ADDRESS:

PHONE:	EMAIL:

DETAILS OF INCIDENT/ACCIDENT

NATURE & EXTENT OF INJURIES:

WHAT ACTION WAS TAKEN: – FIRST AID – AMBULANCE CALLED – HOSPITAL – POLICE – OTHER (PLEASE SPECIFY)

WITNESS(ES)

NAME:	CONTACT:
NAME:	CONTACT:

ACTIONS WHICH COULD HAVE PREVENTED THE INCIDENT

FORM COMPLETED BY:	DATE:
APPROVED BY:	POSITION:
SIGNATURE:	DATE:

INCIDENT / ACCIDENT FORM

INCIDENT DATE:	INCIDENT TIME:
LOCATION:	DATE & TIME REPORTED:

PERSON INJURED / INVOLVED: - EMPLOYEE - VISITOR - GENERAL PUBLIC - CONTRACTOR - OTHER

FULL NAME:

ADDRESS:

PHONE:	EMAIL:

DETAILS OF INCIDENT/ACCIDENT

NATURE & EXTENT OF INJURIES:

WHAT ACTION WAS TAKEN: - FIRST AID - AMBULANCE CALLED - HOSPITAL - POLICE - OTHER (PLEASE SPECIFY)

WITNESS(ES)

NAME:	CONTACT:
NAME:	CONTACT:

ACTIONS WHICH COULD HAVE PREVENTED THE INCIDENT

FORM COMPLETED BY:	DATE:
APPROVED BY:	POSITION:
SIGNATURE:	DATE:

INCIDENT / ACCIDENT FORM

INCIDENT DATE:	INCIDENT TIME:
LOCATION:	DATE & TIME REPORTED:

PERSON INJURED / INVOLVED: – EMPLOYEE – VISITOR – GENERAL PUBLIC – CONTRACTOR – OTHER

FULL NAME:

ADDRESS:

PHONE:	EMAIL:

DETAILS OF INCIDENT/ACCIDENT

NATURE & EXTENT OF INJURIES:

WHAT ACTION WAS TAKEN: – FIRST AID – AMBULANCE CALLED – HOSPITAL – POLICE – OTHER (PLEASE SPECIFY)

WITNESS(ES)

NAME:	CONTACT:
NAME:	CONTACT:

ACTIONS WHICH COULD HAVE PREVENTED THE INCIDENT

FORM COMPLETED BY:	DATE:
APPROVED BY:	POSITION:
SIGNATURE:	DATE:

INCIDENT / ACCIDENT FORM

INCIDENT DATE:	INCIDENT TIME:
LOCATION:	DATE & TIME REPORTED:

PERSON INJURED / INVOLVED: – EMPLOYEE – VISITOR – GENERAL PUBLIC – CONTRACTOR – OTHER

FULL NAME:

ADDRESS:

PHONE:	EMAIL:

DETAILS OF INCIDENT/ACCIDENT

NATURE & EXTENT OF INJURIES:

WHAT ACTION WAS TAKEN: – FIRST AID – AMBULANCE CALLED – HOSPITAL – POLICE – OTHER (PLEASE SPECIFY)

WITNESS(ES)

NAME:	CONTACT:
NAME:	CONTACT:

ACTIONS WHICH COULD HAVE PREVENTED THE INCIDENT

FORM COMPLETED BY:	DATE:
APPROVED BY:	POSITION:
SIGNATURE:	DATE:

INCIDENT / ACCIDENT FORM

INCIDENT DATE:	INCIDENT TIME:
LOCATION:	DATE & TIME REPORTED:

PERSON INJURED / INVOLVED: – EMPLOYEE – VISITOR – GENERAL PUBLIC – CONTRACTOR – OTHER

FULL NAME:

ADDRESS:

PHONE:	EMAIL:

DETAILS OF INCIDENT/ACCIDENT

NATURE & EXTENT OF INJURIES:

WHAT ACTION WAS TAKEN: – FIRST AID – AMBULANCE CALLED – HOSPITAL – POLICE – OTHER (PLEASE SPECIFY)

WITNESS(ES)

NAME:	CONTACT:
NAME:	CONTACT:

ACTIONS WHICH COULD HAVE PREVENTED THE INCIDENT

FORM COMPLETED BY:	DATE:
APPROVED BY:	POSITION:
SIGNATURE:	DATE:

INCIDENT / ACCIDENT FORM

INCIDENT DATE:	INCIDENT TIME:
LOCATION:	DATE & TIME REPORTED:

PERSON INJURED / INVOLVED: – EMPLOYEE – VISITOR – GENERAL PUBLIC – CONTRACTOR – OTHER

FULL NAME:

ADDRESS:

PHONE:	EMAIL:

DETAILS OF INCIDENT/ACCIDENT

NATURE & EXTENT OF INJURIES:

WHAT ACTION WAS TAKEN: – FIRST AID – AMBULANCE CALLED – HOSPITAL – POLICE – OTHER (PLEASE SPECIFY)

WITNESS(ES)

NAME:	CONTACT:
NAME:	CONTACT:

ACTIONS WHICH COULD HAVE PREVENTED THE INCIDENT

FORM COMPLETED BY:	DATE:
APPROVED BY:	POSITION:
SIGNATURE:	DATE:

INCIDENT / ACCIDENT FORM

INCIDENT DATE:	INCIDENT TIME:
LOCATION:	DATE & TIME REPORTED:

PERSON INJURED / INVOLVED: - EMPLOYEE - VISITOR - GENERAL PUBLIC - CONTRACTOR - OTHER

FULL NAME:

ADDRESS:

PHONE:	EMAIL:

DETAILS OF INCIDENT/ACCIDENT

NATURE & EXTENT OF INJURIES:

WHAT ACTION WAS TAKEN: - FIRST AID - AMBULANCE CALLED - HOSPITAL - POLICE - OTHER (PLEASE SPECIFY)

WITNESS(ES)

NAME:	CONTACT:
NAME:	CONTACT:

ACTIONS WHICH COULD HAVE PREVENTED THE INCIDENT

FORM COMPLETED BY:	DATE:
APPROVED BY:	POSITION:
SIGNATURE:	DATE:

INCIDENT / ACCIDENT FORM

INCIDENT DATE:	INCIDENT TIME:
LOCATION:	DATE & TIME REPORTED:

PERSON INJURED / INVOLVED: - EMPLOYEE - VISITOR - GENERAL PUBLIC - CONTRACTOR - OTHER

FULL NAME:

ADDRESS:

PHONE:	EMAIL:

DETAILS OF INCIDENT/ACCIDENT

NATURE & EXTENT OF INJURIES:

WHAT ACTION WAS TAKEN: - FIRST AID - AMBULANCE CALLED - HOSPITAL - POLICE - OTHER (PLEASE SPECIFY)

WITNESS(ES)

NAME:	CONTACT:
NAME:	CONTACT:

ACTIONS WHICH COULD HAVE PREVENTED THE INCIDENT

FORM COMPLETED BY:	DATE:
APPROVED BY:	POSITION:
SIGNATURE:	DATE:

INCIDENT / ACCIDENT FORM

INCIDENT DATE:	INCIDENT TIME:
LOCATION:	DATE & TIME REPORTED:

PERSON INJURED / INVOLVED: – EMPLOYEE – VISITOR – GENERAL PUBLIC – CONTRACTOR – OTHER

FULL NAME:

ADDRESS:

PHONE:	EMAIL:

DETAILS OF INCIDENT/ACCIDENT

NATURE & EXTENT OF INJURIES:

WHAT ACTION WAS TAKEN: – FIRST AID – AMBULANCE CALLED – HOSPITAL – POLICE – OTHER (PLEASE SPECIFY)

WITNESS(ES)

NAME:	CONTACT:
NAME:	CONTACT:

ACTIONS WHICH COULD HAVE PREVENTED THE INCIDENT

FORM COMPLETED BY:	DATE:
APPROVED BY:	POSITION:
SIGNATURE:	DATE:

INCIDENT / ACCIDENT FORM

INCIDENT DATE:	INCIDENT TIME:
LOCATION:	DATE & TIME REPORTED:

PERSON INJURED / INVOLVED: – EMPLOYEE – VISITOR – GENERAL PUBLIC – CONTRACTOR – OTHER

FULL NAME:

ADDRESS:

PHONE:	EMAIL:

DETAILS OF INCIDENT/ACCIDENT

NATURE & EXTENT OF INJURIES:

WHAT ACTION WAS TAKEN: – FIRST AID – AMBULANCE CALLED – HOSPITAL – POLICE – OTHER (PLEASE SPECIFY)

WITNESS(ES)

NAME:	CONTACT:
NAME:	CONTACT:

ACTIONS WHICH COULD HAVE PREVENTED THE INCIDENT

FORM COMPLETED BY:	DATE:
APPROVED BY:	POSITION:
SIGNATURE:	DATE:

INCIDENT / ACCIDENT FORM

INCIDENT DATE:	INCIDENT TIME:
LOCATION:	DATE & TIME REPORTED:

PERSON INJURED / INVOLVED: - EMPLOYEE - VISITOR - GENERAL PUBLIC - CONTRACTOR - OTHER

FULL NAME:

ADDRESS:

PHONE:	EMAIL:

DETAILS OF INCIDENT/ACCIDENT

NATURE & EXTENT OF INJURIES:

WHAT ACTION WAS TAKEN: - FIRST AID - AMBULANCE CALLED - HOSPITAL - POLICE - OTHER (PLEASE SPECIFY)

WITNESS(ES)

NAME:	CONTACT:
NAME:	CONTACT:

ACTIONS WHICH COULD HAVE PREVENTED THE INCIDENT

FORM COMPLETED BY:	DATE:
APPROVED BY:	POSITION:
SIGNATURE:	DATE:

INCIDENT / ACCIDENT FORM

INCIDENT DATE:	INCIDENT TIME:
LOCATION:	DATE & TIME REPORTED:

PERSON INJURED / INVOLVED: – EMPLOYEE – VISITOR – GENERAL PUBLIC – CONTRACTOR – OTHER

FULL NAME:

ADDRESS:

PHONE:	EMAIL:

DETAILS OF INCIDENT/ACCIDENT

NATURE & EXTENT OF INJURIES:

WHAT ACTION WAS TAKEN: – FIRST AID – AMBULANCE CALLED – HOSPITAL – POLICE – OTHER (PLEASE SPECIFY)

WITNESS(ES)

NAME:	CONTACT:
NAME:	CONTACT:

ACTIONS WHICH COULD HAVE PREVENTED THE INCIDENT

FORM COMPLETED BY:	DATE:
APPROVED BY:	POSITION:
SIGNATURE:	DATE:

INCIDENT / ACCIDENT FORM

INCIDENT DATE:	INCIDENT TIME:
LOCATION:	DATE & TIME REPORTED:

PERSON INJURED / INVOLVED: – EMPLOYEE – VISITOR – GENERAL PUBLIC – CONTRACTOR – OTHER

FULL NAME:

ADDRESS:

PHONE:	EMAIL:

DETAILS OF INCIDENT/ACCIDENT

NATURE & EXTENT OF INJURIES:

WHAT ACTION WAS TAKEN: – FIRST AID – AMBULANCE CALLED – HOSPITAL – POLICE – OTHER (PLEASE SPECIFY)

WITNESS(ES)

NAME:	CONTACT:
NAME:	CONTACT:

ACTIONS WHICH COULD HAVE PREVENTED THE INCIDENT

FORM COMPLETED BY:	DATE:
APPROVED BY:	POSITION:
SIGNATURE:	DATE:

INCIDENT / ACCIDENT FORM

INCIDENT DATE:	INCIDENT TIME:
LOCATION:	DATE & TIME REPORTED:

PERSON INJURED / INVOLVED: - EMPLOYEE - VISITOR - GENERAL PUBLIC - CONTRACTOR - OTHER

FULL NAME:

ADDRESS:

PHONE:	EMAIL:

DETAILS OF INCIDENT/ACCIDENT

NATURE & EXTENT OF INJURIES:

WHAT ACTION WAS TAKEN: - FIRST AID - AMBULANCE CALLED - HOSPITAL - POLICE - OTHER (PLEASE SPECIFY)

WITNESS(ES)

NAME:	CONTACT:
NAME:	CONTACT:

ACTIONS WHICH COULD HAVE PREVENTED THE INCIDENT

FORM COMPLETED BY:	DATE:
APPROVED BY:	POSITION:
SIGNATURE:	DATE:

INCIDENT / ACCIDENT FORM

INCIDENT DATE:	INCIDENT TIME:
LOCATION:	DATE & TIME REPORTED:

PERSON INJURED / INVOLVED: – EMPLOYEE – VISITOR – GENERAL PUBLIC – CONTRACTOR – OTHER

FULL NAME:

ADDRESS:

PHONE:	EMAIL:

DETAILS OF INCIDENT/ACCIDENT

NATURE & EXTENT OF INJURIES:

WHAT ACTION WAS TAKEN: – FIRST AID – AMBULANCE CALLED – HOSPITAL – POLICE – OTHER (PLEASE SPECIFY)

WITNESS(ES)

NAME:	CONTACT:
NAME:	CONTACT:

ACTIONS WHICH COULD HAVE PREVENTED THE INCIDENT

FORM COMPLETED BY:	DATE:
APPROVED BY:	POSITION:
SIGNATURE:	DATE:

INCIDENT / ACCIDENT FORM

INCIDENT DATE:	INCIDENT TIME:
LOCATION:	DATE & TIME REPORTED:

PERSON INJURED / INVOLVED: – EMPLOYEE – VISITOR – GENERAL PUBLIC – CONTRACTOR – OTHER

FULL NAME:

ADDRESS:

PHONE:	EMAIL:

DETAILS OF INCIDENT/ACCIDENT

NATURE & EXTENT OF INJURIES:

WHAT ACTION WAS TAKEN: – FIRST AID – AMBULANCE CALLED – HOSPITAL – POLICE – OTHER (PLEASE SPECIFY)

WITNESS(ES)

NAME:	CONTACT:
NAME:	CONTACT:

ACTIONS WHICH COULD HAVE PREVENTED THE INCIDENT

FORM COMPLETED BY:	DATE:
APPROVED BY:	POSITION:
SIGNATURE:	DATE:

INCIDENT / ACCIDENT FORM

INCIDENT DATE:	INCIDENT TIME:
LOCATION:	DATE & TIME REPORTED:

PERSON INJURED / INVOLVED: – EMPLOYEE – VISITOR – GENERAL PUBLIC – CONTRACTOR – OTHER

FULL NAME:

ADDRESS:

PHONE:	EMAIL:

DETAILS OF INCIDENT/ACCIDENT

NATURE & EXTENT OF INJURIES:

WHAT ACTION WAS TAKEN: – FIRST AID – AMBULANCE CALLED – HOSPITAL – POLICE – OTHER (PLEASE SPECIFY)

WITNESS(ES)

NAME:	CONTACT:
NAME:	CONTACT:

ACTIONS WHICH COULD HAVE PREVENTED THE INCIDENT

FORM COMPLETED BY:	DATE:
APPROVED BY:	POSITION:
SIGNATURE:	DATE:

INCIDENT / ACCIDENT FORM

INCIDENT DATE:	INCIDENT TIME:
LOCATION:	DATE & TIME REPORTED:

PERSON INJURED / INVOLVED: - EMPLOYEE - VISITOR - GENERAL PUBLIC - CONTRACTOR - OTHER

FULL NAME:

ADDRESS:

PHONE:	EMAIL:

DETAILS OF INCIDENT/ACCIDENT

NATURE & EXTENT OF INJURIES:

WHAT ACTION WAS TAKEN: - FIRST AID - AMBULANCE CALLED - HOSPITAL - POLICE - OTHER (PLEASE SPECIFY)

WITNESS(ES)

NAME:	CONTACT:
NAME:	CONTACT:

ACTIONS WHICH COULD HAVE PREVENTED THE INCIDENT

FORM COMPLETED BY:	DATE:
APPROVED BY:	POSITION:
SIGNATURE:	DATE:

INCIDENT / ACCIDENT FORM

INCIDENT DATE:	INCIDENT TIME:
LOCATION:	DATE & TIME REPORTED:

PERSON INJURED / INVOLVED: - EMPLOYEE - VISITOR - GENERAL PUBLIC - CONTRACTOR - OTHER

FULL NAME:

ADDRESS:

PHONE:	EMAIL:

DETAILS OF INCIDENT/ACCIDENT

NATURE & EXTENT OF INJURIES:

WHAT ACTION WAS TAKEN: - FIRST AID - AMBULANCE CALLED - HOSPITAL - POLICE - OTHER (PLEASE SPECIFY)

WITNESS(ES)

NAME:	CONTACT:
NAME:	CONTACT:

ACTIONS WHICH COULD HAVE PREVENTED THE INCIDENT

FORM COMPLETED BY:	DATE:
APPROVED BY:	POSITION:
SIGNATURE:	DATE:

INCIDENT / ACCIDENT FORM

INCIDENT DATE:	INCIDENT TIME:
LOCATION:	DATE & TIME REPORTED:

PERSON INJURED / INVOLVED: – EMPLOYEE – VISITOR – GENERAL PUBLIC – CONTRACTOR – OTHER

FULL NAME:

ADDRESS:

PHONE:	EMAIL:

DETAILS OF INCIDENT/ACCIDENT

NATURE & EXTENT OF INJURIES:

WHAT ACTION WAS TAKEN: – FIRST AID – AMBULANCE CALLED – HOSPITAL – POLICE – OTHER (PLEASE SPECIFY)

WITNESS(ES)

NAME:	CONTACT:
NAME:	CONTACT:

ACTIONS WHICH COULD HAVE PREVENTED THE INCIDENT

FORM COMPLETED BY:	DATE:
APPROVED BY:	POSITION:
SIGNATURE:	DATE:

INCIDENT / ACCIDENT FORM

INCIDENT DATE:	INCIDENT TIME:
LOCATION:	DATE & TIME REPORTED:

PERSON INJURED / INVOLVED: – EMPLOYEE – VISITOR – GENERAL PUBLIC – CONTRACTOR – OTHER

FULL NAME:

ADDRESS:

PHONE:	EMAIL:

DETAILS OF INCIDENT/ACCIDENT

NATURE & EXTENT OF INJURIES:

WHAT ACTION WAS TAKEN: – FIRST AID – AMBULANCE CALLED – HOSPITAL – POLICE – OTHER (PLEASE SPECIFY)

WITNESS(ES)

NAME:	CONTACT:
NAME:	CONTACT:

ACTIONS WHICH COULD HAVE PREVENTED THE INCIDENT

FORM COMPLETED BY:	DATE:
APPROVED BY:	POSITION:
SIGNATURE:	DATE:

INCIDENT / ACCIDENT FORM

INCIDENT DATE:	INCIDENT TIME:
LOCATION:	DATE & TIME REPORTED:

PERSON INJURED / INVOLVED: – EMPLOYEE – VISITOR – GENERAL PUBLIC – CONTRACTOR – OTHER

FULL NAME:

ADDRESS:

PHONE:	EMAIL:

DETAILS OF INCIDENT/ACCIDENT

NATURE & EXTENT OF INJURIES:

WHAT ACTION WAS TAKEN: – FIRST AID – AMBULANCE CALLED – HOSPITAL – POLICE – OTHER (PLEASE SPECIFY)

WITNESS(ES)

NAME:	CONTACT:
NAME:	CONTACT:

ACTIONS WHICH COULD HAVE PREVENTED THE INCIDENT

FORM COMPLETED BY:	DATE:
APPROVED BY:	POSITION:
SIGNATURE:	DATE:

INCIDENT / ACCIDENT FORM

INCIDENT DATE:	INCIDENT TIME:
LOCATION:	DATE & TIME REPORTED:
PERSON INJURED / INVOLVED: – EMPLOYEE – VISITOR – GENERAL PUBLIC – CONTRACTOR – OTHER	
FULL NAME:	
ADDRESS:	
PHONE:	EMAIL:

DETAILS OF INCIDENT/ACCIDENT

NATURE & EXTENT OF INJURIES:

WHAT ACTION WAS TAKEN: – FIRST AID – AMBULANCE CALLED – HOSPITAL – POLICE – OTHER (PLEASE SPECIFY)

WITNESS(ES)

NAME:	CONTACT:
NAME:	CONTACT:

ACTIONS WHICH COULD HAVE PREVENTED THE INCIDENT

FORM COMPLETED BY:	DATE:
APPROVED BY:	POSITION:
SIGNATURE:	DATE:

INCIDENT / ACCIDENT FORM

INCIDENT DATE:	INCIDENT TIME:
LOCATION:	DATE & TIME REPORTED:

PERSON INJURED / INVOLVED: – EMPLOYEE – VISITOR – GENERAL PUBLIC – CONTRACTOR – OTHER

FULL NAME:

ADDRESS:

PHONE:	EMAIL:

DETAILS OF INCIDENT/ACCIDENT

NATURE & EXTENT OF INJURIES:

WHAT ACTION WAS TAKEN: – FIRST AID – AMBULANCE CALLED – HOSPITAL – POLICE – OTHER (PLEASE SPECIFY)

WITNESS(ES)

NAME:	CONTACT:
NAME:	CONTACT:

ACTIONS WHICH COULD HAVE PREVENTED THE INCIDENT

FORM COMPLETED BY:	DATE:
APPROVED BY:	POSITION:
SIGNATURE:	DATE:

INCIDENT / ACCIDENT FORM

INCIDENT DATE:	INCIDENT TIME:
LOCATION:	DATE & TIME REPORTED:

PERSON INJURED / INVOLVED: - EMPLOYEE - VISITOR - GENERAL PUBLIC - CONTRACTOR - OTHER

FULL NAME:

ADDRESS:

PHONE:	EMAIL:

DETAILS OF INCIDENT/ACCIDENT

NATURE & EXTENT OF INJURIES:

WHAT ACTION WAS TAKEN: - FIRST AID - AMBULANCE CALLED - HOSPITAL - POLICE - OTHER (PLEASE SPECIFY)

WITNESS(ES)

NAME:	CONTACT:
NAME:	CONTACT:

ACTIONS WHICH COULD HAVE PREVENTED THE INCIDENT

FORM COMPLETED BY:	DATE:
APPROVED BY:	POSITION:
SIGNATURE:	DATE:

INCIDENT / ACCIDENT FORM

INCIDENT DATE:	INCIDENT TIME:
LOCATION:	DATE & TIME REPORTED:

PERSON INJURED / INVOLVED: - EMPLOYEE - VISITOR - GENERAL PUBLIC - CONTRACTOR - OTHER

FULL NAME:

ADDRESS:

PHONE:	EMAIL:

DETAILS OF INCIDENT/ACCIDENT

NATURE & EXTENT OF INJURIES:

WHAT ACTION WAS TAKEN: - FIRST AID - AMBULANCE CALLED - HOSPITAL - POLICE - OTHER (PLEASE SPECIFY)

WITNESS(ES)

NAME:	CONTACT:
NAME:	CONTACT:

ACTIONS WHICH COULD HAVE PREVENTED THE INCIDENT

FORM COMPLETED BY:	DATE:
APPROVED BY:	POSITION:
SIGNATURE:	DATE:

INCIDENT / ACCIDENT FORM

INCIDENT DATE:	INCIDENT TIME:
LOCATION:	DATE & TIME REPORTED:

PERSON INJURED / INVOLVED: - EMPLOYEE - VISITOR - GENERAL PUBLIC - CONTRACTOR - OTHER

FULL NAME:

ADDRESS:

PHONE:	EMAIL:

DETAILS OF INCIDENT/ACCIDENT

NATURE & EXTENT OF INJURIES:

WHAT ACTION WAS TAKEN: - FIRST AID - AMBULANCE CALLED - HOSPITAL - POLICE - OTHER (PLEASE SPECIFY)

WITNESS(ES)

NAME:	CONTACT:
NAME:	CONTACT:

ACTIONS WHICH COULD HAVE PREVENTED THE INCIDENT

FORM COMPLETED BY:	DATE:
APPROVED BY:	POSITION:
SIGNATURE:	DATE:

INCIDENT / ACCIDENT FORM

INCIDENT DATE:	INCIDENT TIME:
LOCATION:	DATE & TIME REPORTED:

PERSON INJURED / INVOLVED: – EMPLOYEE – VISITOR – GENERAL PUBLIC – CONTRACTOR – OTHER

FULL NAME:

ADDRESS:

PHONE:	EMAIL:

DETAILS OF INCIDENT/ACCIDENT

NATURE & EXTENT OF INJURIES:

WHAT ACTION WAS TAKEN: – FIRST AID – AMBULANCE CALLED – HOSPITAL – POLICE – OTHER (PLEASE SPECIFY)

WITNESS(ES)

NAME:	CONTACT:
NAME:	CONTACT:

ACTIONS WHICH COULD HAVE PREVENTED THE INCIDENT

FORM COMPLETED BY:	DATE:
APPROVED BY:	POSITION:
SIGNATURE:	DATE:

INCIDENT / ACCIDENT FORM

INCIDENT DATE:	INCIDENT TIME:
LOCATION:	DATE & TIME REPORTED:

PERSON INJURED / INVOLVED: – EMPLOYEE – VISITOR – GENERAL PUBLIC – CONTRACTOR – OTHER

FULL NAME:

ADDRESS:

PHONE:	EMAIL:

DETAILS OF INCIDENT/ACCIDENT

NATURE & EXTENT OF INJURIES:

WHAT ACTION WAS TAKEN: – FIRST AID – AMBULANCE CALLED – HOSPITAL – POLICE – OTHER (PLEASE SPECIFY)

WITNESS(ES)

NAME:	CONTACT:
NAME:	CONTACT:

ACTIONS WHICH COULD HAVE PREVENTED THE INCIDENT

FORM COMPLETED BY:	DATE:
APPROVED BY:	POSITION:
SIGNATURE:	DATE:

Printed in Great Britain
by Amazon